# CONFERENCE

by

L. LANDOUZY. M. D.

Professor of the Laënnec's Medical Clinic

at the University of Paris

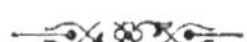

# MONT-DORE

(Puy-de-Dôme)

## HYDROMINERAL STATION

## AND HIGH AIR CURE

Papier, Gravure et Impression

Louis GEISLER,

aux Châtelles, par Raon-l'Étape (Vosges).

—

1908

First Floor

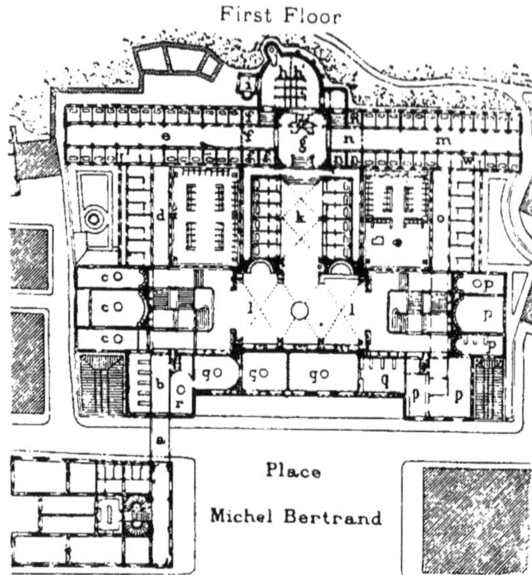


Thermal springs : 1 Rigny, 2 Madeleine, 3 Ramon, 4 Boyer, 5 Pigeon, 6 des Chanteurs, 7 du Panthéon, 8 Boyer-Bertrand, 9 de l'Angle, 10 du Pavillon, 11 Cesar.

Hyperthermal baths : l, g, h. — Gallery for temperate baths and douches : m, o, k, d, e — Inhalations rooms : p, q, c, Z. — Steam douches : R. — Cabins for gargling : T, N. — Rhinopharyngeal irrigations : S, M. — Hall for foot-baths : J, O.—Gaseous nasal pulverisations : f, n. — Hydrotherapia : K, Q. — Administration : C, D, E.

Ground Floor

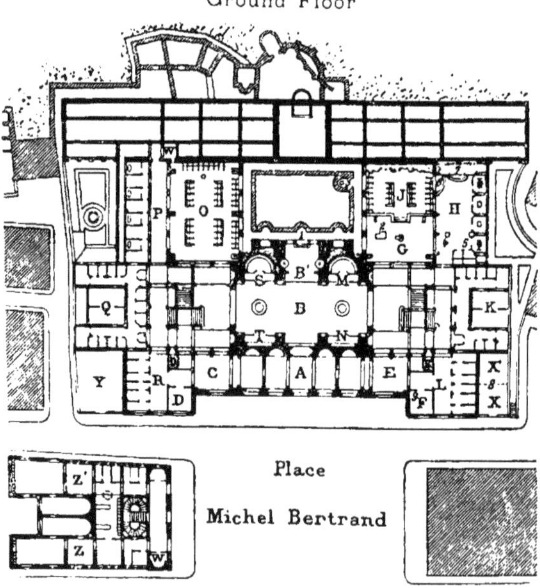

*Summary of the Conference :*

# MONT-DORE

(PUY-DE-DOMF)

## HYDROMINERAL STATION AND HIGH-AIR CURE

HYPERTHERMAL WATERS.
GASEOUS AND ALCALINE.
BICARBONATED MIXED.
ARSENICAL, SILICIOUS, AND FERRUGINEOUS.



| | | |
|---|---|---|
| **MONT-DORE CURE** | PRINCIPAL | *High-Air*<br>*Drink,*<br>*Inhalations.*<br>*Hyperthermal baths in running Water.* |
| | ANNEXED | *Rhinopharyngeal Irrigations and Pulverisations*<br>*Gaseous nasal douches.*<br>*Temperate baths and Foot baths*<br>*Liquid and steam Douches,*<br>*Warm and cold Hydrotherapy.* |

### THOSE AMENABLE TO :

*A*) THE DIATHESIC SPECIALISATIONS ARE :

1° The patients presenting the neuro-arthritic reactional form
2° Hereditary neuro-arthritic persons.
3° Certain Diabetic patients threatened or affected with respiratory troubles;

*B*) THE FONCTIONAL SPECIALISATIONS :

1° Patients suffering from respiratory troubles, of a more or less catarrhal form, and especially if spasmodic or congestive:
— Whatever the local disorders may be, whether rhinopharyngeal, laryngeal, tracheo-bronchial, pulmonary or pleural.
— whether it be cases of diathesic irritation, either professional or accidental;
— whether it may be in cases of inflammation, more or less stationary, in the train of infectious diseases (influenza, measles, whooping-cough, and in certain cases tuberculosis).

2° Children who, through their personal antecedents or inheritance are threatened or affected with respiratory disorders.

3° Certian eczematic patients with manifestations sometimes on the skin and sometimes in the respiratory organs.

4° Persons affected with arthralgia, neuralgia, alternating or not with respiratory troubles

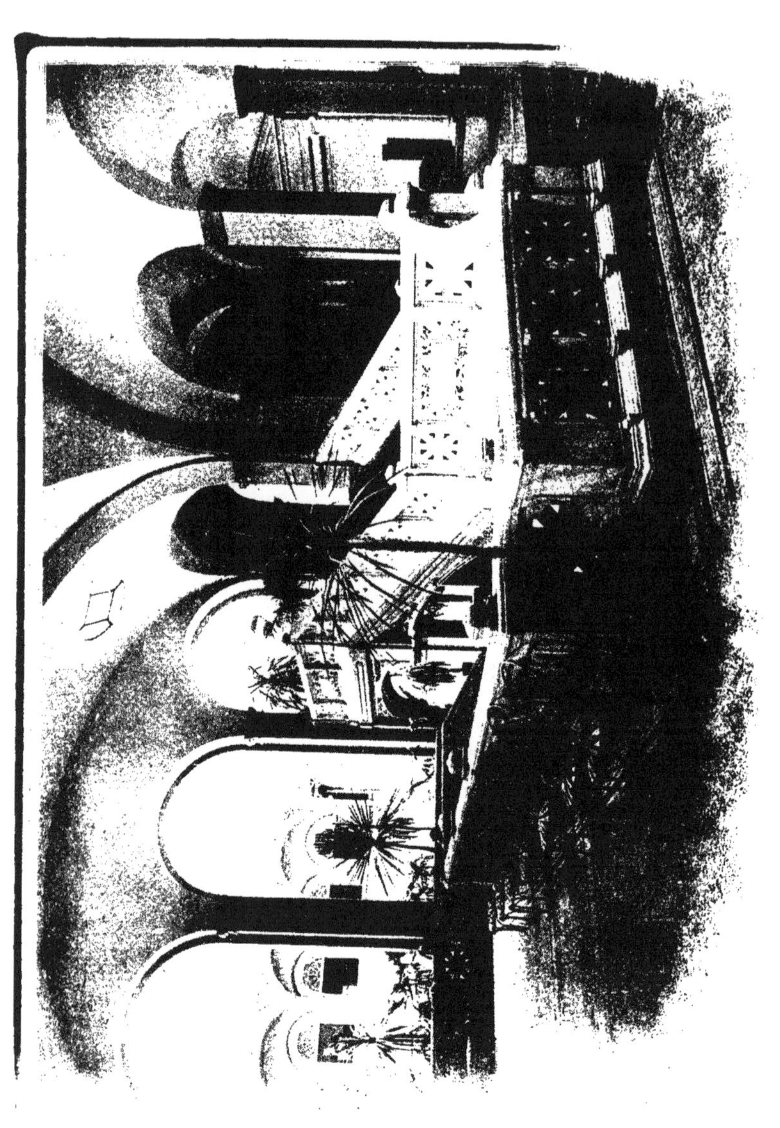

# MONT-DORE (1)

Gentlemen,

It is with the greatest satisfaction that I find myself again at Mont-Dore with the V. E. M. (2), not only because as six years ago, we are again favoured by such lovely weather, which allows us to enjoy the rugged beauty of the volcanoes of Auvergne and to appreciate the feeling of well being afforded by the pure light air of these mountains, but especially because from the point of view of Therapeutic study, which is the aim of our journey, this station is really one of the most interesting and instructive as well as one of those on which the practising doctors will most rely.

The place is one of the most important from the fact that here the *hydro-mineral cure* is *intimately associated with the high-air cure*, and also because the efficacious combination of two physiotherapic modalities, the convergence of two distinct curative powers is here realised, as I already remarked some years ago to the partisans of the anivocal treatment of the pulmonary tuberculous patients in a Sanatorium.

Mont-Dore is curious for the age of its use, revealed by the vestiges of wooden pools, dating from before the Gallo Roman epoch. It is also curious for the *Therapeutic importance of its functional specialisation*, originally defined and *clearly limited*.

Mont-Dore is moreover, recommended to physicians and patients on account of the transformation undergone since the last fifteen years in its installment, fitted up with every comfort and in perfect accordance with modern sanitary requirements.

It is sufficient to speak of the extreme interest attached to the study of:

(1°) The Mont-Dore medicament,

(2°) The Mont-Dore medication,

(3°) The patients an expert selection of whom do justice to this station.

---

(1) Conference made in the form of an *Object Lesson of practical Thermal Therapeutics* in the great hall of the Casino of Mont-Dore on September 5 th 1904, by professor Landouzy, Scientific director of the " Voyages d'Etudes Medicales " of the hydro-mineral, navy, and climatic stations of France.

The sixth of these V. E. M. organised since 1899 by Doctor Carron de la Carriere took more than a hundred of these from all parts of the world, from September 3 rd to 15 th to visit the stations in the centre of France and Auvergne : Lamotte-Beuvron, Neris, Evaux, Mont-Dore, Saint-Nectaire, La Bourboule, Vic-sur-Cere and Lioran Royat Chatel-Guyon Vichy, Bourbon-l'Archambault Bourbon-Lancy, Saint-Honoré-les-Bains, Pougues.

(2) Conference made September 1899 published 1899 as a sumary : *Report given of the V. E. M. to the stations in the centre of France* (G. CARRÉ et NAUD, publishers, Paris 1900; and the *Medical Review of Mont-Dore*, No 1 April 1905).

(3) *Simple and associated Cure* (G. CARRÉ et C. NAUD publishers, Paris 1899 and *Medical Press*, No 42 May 27 th 1899).

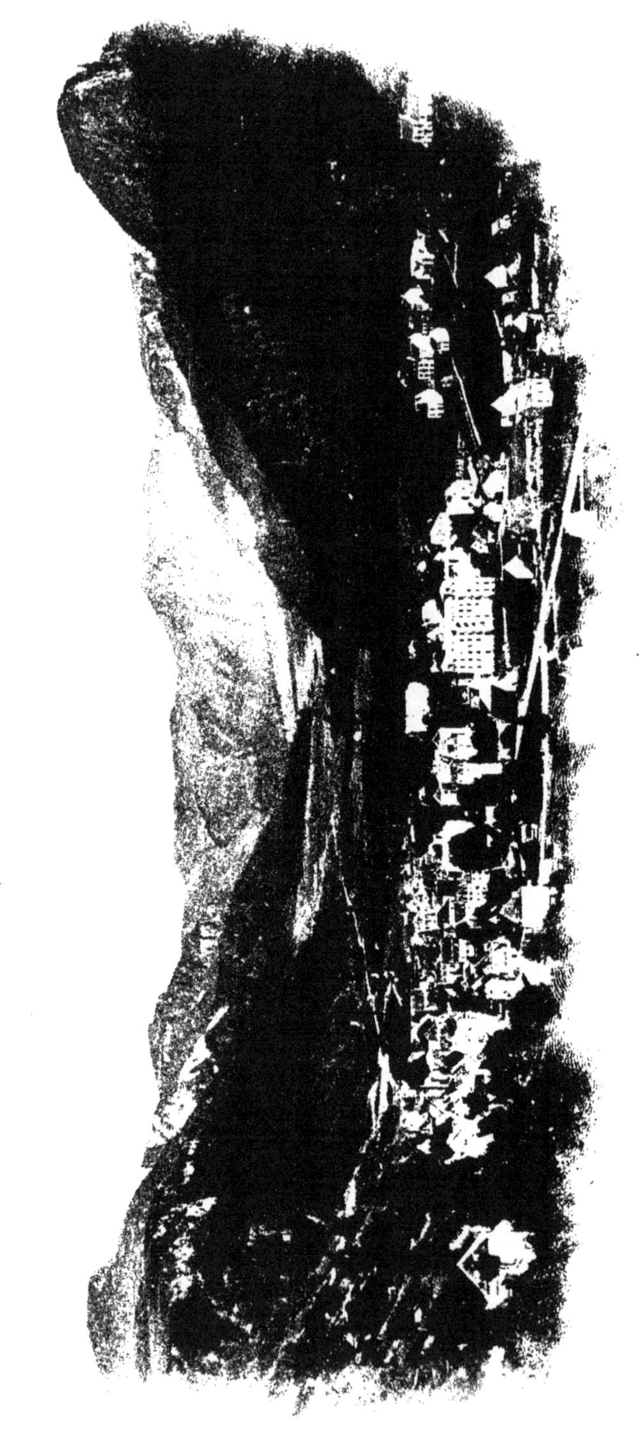

# The Mont-Dore Medicament

I

A few words to begin with, on the TOPOGRAPHY of this mountain station :

The Terminus Station of one of the branches of the Orleans railway, Mont-Dore at 10 hours from Paris, 16 hours from Brussels and 19 hours from London, communicates with the Capital by the express of the Orleans C$^{o}$. At the stations of Clermont and of Neussargues, the line is united to that of the express of the P.-L.-M. C$^{o}$ to Switzerland and Italy, or joins the branches of the South.

Situated at 3,446 feet above the sea-level in the very centre of volcanoes, towards the South West of the department of Puy-de-Dôme, the station leans against the basaltic basis of the table land of Angle, in the valley of the Dordogne river, which is overlooked on the South by the Peak of Sancy (6186) and on the North is barred by the Puy Gros (4887).

On the West, the Capucin tableland (4100) forms in the midst of a most lovely forest of hoary pines and firs, a natural almost horizontal park, where the patients spend the greater part of the afternoon, and which they can reach in five minutes by the first electric funicular railway built in France.

Mont-Dore is therefore with Escaldas (4448 feet) and Baréges (4040) both Pyreneesan sulphurous stations, one of the three highest thermal stations of France.

II

If the Mont-Dore waters, which resemble that of La Bourboule in some of its components, is less strongly loaded with arsenic, it has, and very justly too, at least an equal reputation. At all times Mont-Dore has been famous for its SPECIAL ACTION ON THE RESPIRATORY ORGANS, just as La Bourboule, a more recent station, has been since its creation in the middle of last century for its special effect on the skin.

With regard to the *way in which to consider and study the* MEDICINAL VIRTUES *the therapeutic properties peculiar to the Mineral waters*, Mont-Dore affords us a new example which supports the fact I have many times insisted on, chiefly at Ax-les-Thermes, and to which I again wish to call your attention :

" To the ancient classifications of Medical Matter, taking their remedy from the three kingdoms Animal, Mineral, and Vegetable, we must, as I already said last year, add a fourth, namely, the *Organic mineral* kingdom in which we find the Thermal waters, taken at the spout, these *mineral lymphs* which with their organic combinations as well as their thermo-electric state, resemble so much the natural serums, the lymphs that bathe our tissues.

Really in general Therapeutics as well as in Pharmacodinamics, the *organised* metallic hydrates, that are the thermal Springs, should be distinguished from the remedies of which the substance is drawn from the Medical Mineral Matter of our ancient Pharmacopoeia.

What comparison of phisico chemical constitution, what parity of statics and of dynamics, in fact can be made between thermal water, whether sulphorous or arsenical or bi-carbonated, drunk at the source or taken in a bath of running water, and a solute of sulphur of potassium, arseniate of soda or Vichy Salts prepared in an Apothecary's laboratory ?

However justified the interest taken in the contributions successively brought through Chemistry to the most intimate knowledge of the constituent elements of this medicinal lymphe may be, the mineralogical science only just begins to notice the intermolecular changes, the true organic mutations, which during their ascending course, interpret the vitality of thermal springs. Of the notation of the respective weights of the divers mineral principles found in thermal water, can one even to-day conclude on the existence and degree of its radio-activity ? Can one judge of its electro-energetic capacity ?

And — since the Mont-Dore water is precisely the first organic mineral medecine in which Scoutteten discovered and followed the deviations of the galvanometric needle — I may well be allowed to remind you herewith, that it is not to the chemist's scales but to the investigation of the Mineral water, well studied and considered in all its complexity as a living organism that we owe the discovery of Magnetic energy, amongst the different kinds of energy, shown in the vitality of the Thermal spring.

As to the manifestations of its phisiological activity, *in presence of the human reagent*, as to its therapeutic character respecting the diathesic alterations and functional disorders, I really do not think you will even be able to perceive them in the simple inspection of the divers chemical elements which form the mineralisation, relatively weak, of the Mont-Dore water.

Here, as in the other Stations, the Empiricism had, in times immemorial, made known the particular medicinal properties of the Springs. This we learn from Michael Bertrand, whose studies on policlinics contributed so much to prove the *special action* of the Mont-Dore waters. « Some poor sick people, he says, who were living in the neighbourhood of the springs were the first to profit by and to speak of their virtues. Their story was as simple as they themselves, and as true as the action of the remedy. Thus began and spread, little by little and without intrigue, the fame of our Thermal waters ».

We find far back in the Mont-Dore history, manyp recious documents speaking of the first Therapeutic uses made of these springs and the vapours that rise from them; giving very precise information left there in the fifth century by Sidonius Apollinary, and according to him the traditional application of these waters to the respiratory organs appears to remount much farther back still.

With regard to the antiquity of the Specialisation of Mont-Dore, it may be interesting here to cast a glance at the bust of the old *Roman*, the shape of which is well worthy of our attention. With his raised shoulders, his arched breast-bone, his curved breast, his projecting eyes, Is he not represented as a person suffering from asthmatic emphysema ? With his short neck from the remounting of the thorax ? Is not this the impression made by that old statue of basaltic stone, that now decorates the large halls of the modern Establishment, just as it adorned that of the luxurious Gallo Romans many centuries ago. If we may be allowed to discuss, from an archeological point of view, the meaning of the spheroidal weapon placed on his right and now considered to be an attribute of Arian origin symbolising his recovered strength, it must be remarked that, from a medical point of view, amongst the numerous statues discovered in the ancient hydropoles in France and abroad, this is the only one to which the sculptor who undertook the decoration of the Thermae has given the characteristic features of a man suffering from broncho emphysema ?

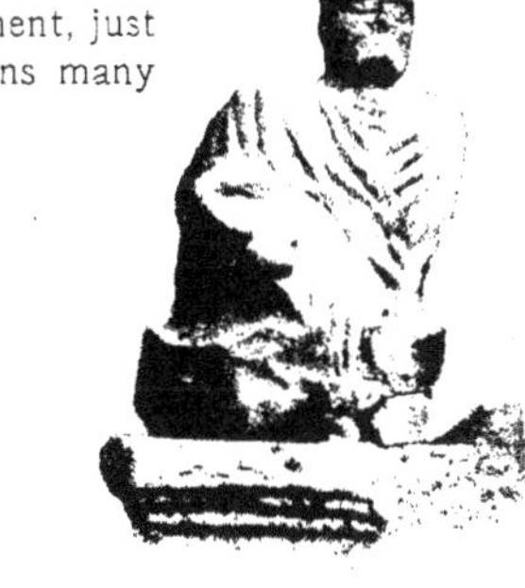

On account of its medical specialisation and value, such as were discovered in the time of the old Empire, and such as were precisely stated by the observations of modern clinics, such as we are about to see confirmed in the study of the hydro-mineral medicamentation; on account of the numerous medical requirements to which it can give ample satisfaction, as well as through the qualities of its installment and accessories, Mont-Dore deserves, with its therapeutic qualities, (which are as peculiar to itself as they are important) to be reckoned amongst the first class hydro-mineral stations of the world.

## III

The study of the Mont-Dore station is also instructive, as I have already remarked, on account of its HYGIENIC RENOVATION : the Establishment at the time of its restoration in 1890 was the first to inaugurate the reign of asepsie joined to comfort, and since then thanks to the initiative of its inhabitants the principles of modern prophylaxie have been applied not only in the public buildings, the new villas and first class hotels, but also in the older habitations in which one now finds every security that scientific disinfection can give.

Through the improvement in its municipal service, the formation of bands of disinfecting men, the extension and perfection of its sewerage system, and the individual efforts of the hotel keepers, the station is compelled to reassure the public of any fear that the discovery of Kock's bacillus might have thrown on some of the thermal stations, discrediting them momentarily, even though they were the most justly famous for their special therapeutic action, such as Mont-Dore, Allevard, Eaux-Bonnes. With all the hygienic securities which Mont-Dore offers to-day to the divers and numerous bathers, it is placed above all suspicion. It realises the prediction I made in 1895 when I said that the stations frequented by tuberculous patients would be the places where one would be the safest from the bacillary infection, just as we know to-day that the best place to safe-guard one's self againts the strepto-coccic contamination is in the Maternity hospitals.

## IV

Let us now consider the medical matter itself, the MINERAL WATER, of which we shall presently study the divers processes of employment.

It is inside the thermal establishment (lined with waterproof tiles and intersected by canals, a veritable pattern of aseptic installation, which after each morning service is used to wash the floors with running water) that, spouting directly from the volcanic trachytis chimneys without any pipes whatever and sheltered from the dust by their glass cages, the 12 **Mont-Dore springs** flow, pouring forth about 200.000 gallons a day; the temperature on leaving the rock varies from 100 to 115° F. excepting the **Marguerite** spring, used sometimes as table water, cold gaseous and acidulated. The Mont-Dore water, heavily loaded with gases of which the most abundant is carbonic acid, flows from the ground boiling and forms on the surface an iridescent pellicule principally of silica, which leaves on the sides of the basin a deposit reminding one of certain kinds of agate.

The water, which is thus drunk in a living state, immediately on leaving the spouts presenting itself with the full activity of its molecular mutations, with all its organic mobility, its chemical, magnetic electric or radio-active powers that make of it a real medicinal lymph, flows into the glass transparent and clear or down through the tubes for bottleing.

Exported, the patients can, in any part of the world, continue or recommence the cure at home, at opportune intervals, and contribute to the just fame of Mont-Dore.

I must mention apart the **FELIX** spring, belonging to a different regimen, which bubbles up at about 2 kilometers from the Establishment and which, richer in bi-carbonate of lythium, is often successfully prescribed in case of urinary gravel, as would be the Martigny water, which contains the same quantity of lithyum.

As to the springs spouting in the Establishment, the **Chanteurs, Madeleine, César,** and **Ramond** are chiefly used for drinking purposes, and the **Panthéon** and **Pavillon** springs for hyperthermal hip-baths in running water. They all present a global mineralisation of from 30 to 45 grains of which 15 of bi-carbonates, and varying little according to the spout from which it springs.

| | Grains | | |
|---|---|---|---|
| Bi-carbonate of soda | 8.27 | to | 8.37 |
| — chalk | 4.19 | — | 5.58 |
| — magnesia | 2.51 | — | 2.71 |
| — potash. | 0.32 | — | 0.47 |
| — iron. | 0.30 | — | 0.49 |
| — lythium | 0.01 | — | 0.12 |
| Cloride of soda. | 5.49 | — | 0.57 |
| Silica. | 2.39 | — | 2.59 |
| Sulphate of soda | 1.02 | — | 1.18 |
| Alum. | 0.08 | — | 1.16 |
| Arsenate of soda | 0.01 | — | 0.01 |
| Borax | traces | | |
| Iodine | | | |
| Bromure | | | |
| Florure | | | |
| Oxide of manganese. | signs | | |
| — coesium. | | | |
| — rubidium | | | |

What we must retain from this chemical analysis is that we are speaking of a water feebly *alcaline, gaseous, bicarbonated, arsenical, ferruginous* and *silicious*, with this peculiarity that the Mont-Dore water contains more silica than any other of the French waters.

With regard to the gases given out spontaneously by the springs, according to the analysis made by Parmentier, 100 volumes contain 99.50 of Carbonic Acid, 0,49 of Nitrogen, 0.01 of Argon and no traces of Oxigen.

On evaporating in vacuum distilled water into which these gases have been mixed, together with the sulphuric acid, we obtain a weak saline residuum formed chiefly of silica, bromures and chlorides.

On ending this *anatomic* study of the Mont-Dore water, I must once more remind you that it is an organic mineral medicine and before leaving the domains of the laboratory, You will note, that there, it already shows its vitality in the divers phenomenae that cause the various effects of the energetic power with which it is gifted.

We must therefore observe, amongst the accumulated energies, the very-special affinity shown in the Mont-Dore water, when exposed to the open air, with regard to the oxigen of which it absorbs according to MM. Coignart and Bretet ten times as much as does distilled water.

So it is that — without stopping to speak again of Scutteten's galvanic experience — I must point out the spectroscopic rays of the helium in the gases which escape from the springs, showing their radio-activity, recently discovered by M. Currie.

However important and suggestive may be our knowledge of the statics and dynamics of the Mont-Dore springs, and on their chemical properties, you will understand that here, as in many other stations it would never be sufficient to evolve the indications, to determine the special diathesic and functional action, which has made the worldly fame of Mont-Dore.

Ought I again to repeat that the thermal special action, the therapeutic indications already mentioned, as well as the hydro-mineral cure opportunely applied, are really the result of sagacious practice and ingenious experience of our fellow doctors of the stations, rather than the result of inquiries and analysis made by chemists.

Without depreciating the study of thermo-chemistry, without despising the therapeutic premises due to the analysis in a laboratory, I may assert that our patients, through the relief, comfort and recovery obtained from the seasons spent at Mont-Dore, have, from the time of Sidonius Appolinary, from Dr Bertrand down to the polyclinic of our fellow members, who do honour to the Establishment, the most and the best shown the reality of the special effect of Mont-Dore.

Hence the fact that the members of the V. E. M. so often hear me repeat what I have taken from a saying found in our old pharmacopiae and adapted to the hydro-mineral medication : *Naturam aquarum affectus et curationes ostendunt.*

It is not surprising, after all, — since we are speaking of waters of action solicited by medicine and of reaction produced by a patient — that it is our fellow members rather than the chemists who have shown us how and how many different therapeutic effects can be obtained from the springs of peculiar mineralisation and original composition. Remark here that I do not confuse mineralisation with composition : the composition of a water spring comprises really many other things besides the nature of its chemical elements, for it comprises the ordination of these elements as well as their electric and thermal state, their mutation, their radio-activity, etc.

How many graduated therapeutic effects are obtained at Mont-Dore by the use of the great mineral and thermic scale ! What a variety of cures made by the patients, some coming here, in large numbers, for respiratory diseases, others for neuralgia, articular pains, diabetis !

# The Mont-Dore Treatment

We must now consider the DIFFERENT MODES OF EMPLOYMENT of the medicament and THEIR CORRESPONDING EFFECT on bathers and drinkers.

I

I will not however stay here to speak of the MEDICATION ANNEXED to the Mont-Dore cure, such as **common hydrotheropia**, nor even of the **temperate baths** composed of fresh water and mineral water employed for their sedative influence nor of the **liquid mineral douches** or **steam douches**, employed either as revulsive measures or applied locally as a resolvent, used especially in the treatment of articular affections.

Neither will I stop to speak of CERTAIN LOCALISED APPLICATIONS OF THE MONT-DORE CURE, notwithstanding their great therapeutic value, such as these of the gases spontaneously emitted by the springs and collected according to their employment in the form of **gaseous nasal douches** of which the local action (anaesthetic and constringent) is generally lasting and is used with success in certain cases of rhinorrhia.

The *mineral water is also applied directly to the mocous membranes by* **gargles,** *rhinapharyngeal* **irrigations** or **pulverisations** in **larynx** and throat on which it has a slight astringent and tonic effect.

It is sufficient for me to remind you of how often the first aerial tubes are infected and how the latter interfere with the physiological or pathological set of respiratory organs, for you to see the importance of the topical application of a medicine, now anaesthetic and sedative, now tonic and abstergant, assuring or restablishing the functional integrity of the superior aerial mucous membranes.

II

I am anxious to study with you most especially the THREE PRINCIPAL MODES OF EMPLOYMENT of the Mont-Dore waters, that with the high-air cure impress on the medication its real characteristic features. and to explain to you, little more or less as I did six years ago, the processes of :

1° **Drinking;**
2° **Mineral baths** (hyperthermal hip-baths, foot baths, hand baths).
3° **Inhalations.**

The **Drinking** process at Mont-Dore is of very great importance : by this cure alone numerous patients have experienced great improvement. Of a slight styptic taste, the Mont-Dore water introduced into the stomach increases the secretion of hydrocloric acid; — although it does not greatly increase the diuresis, it provokes regularly a notable discharge of uric acid; the loss then diminishes in azoted waste and in imperfect oxide produce; — rather astringent, except in idiosyncrasic intolerance, it appears to eliminate chiefly through the mucous membranes of respiratory organs, on which it acts, *mutatis mutandis*, like a balsam drug.

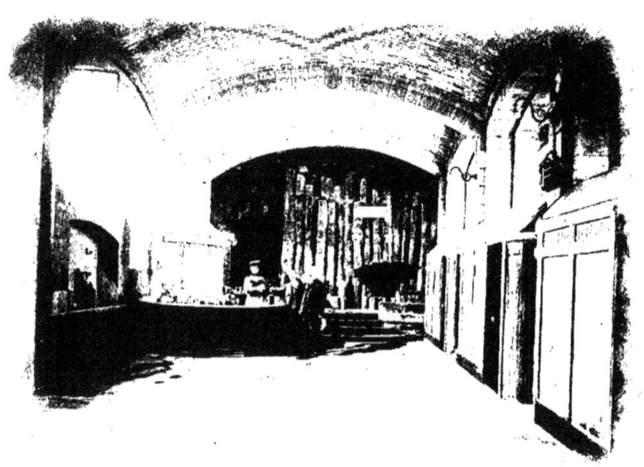

Besides this, in cases of diabetis it generally decreases, in a very notable and persistent manner, the rate of glycosuria.

Such are, shortly summed up, the observations noted with regard to the ingestion of the Mont-Dore water, as well by the doctors who have experimented on themselves with it as by the patients treated exclusively in this manner.

To the drinking cure (without the help of hyperthermal baths or inhalations) we can put down the general reconstituant effect felt by the patient, as well as the decongestive and sedative action, objectively and subjectively marked, on the whole of the respiratory apparatus.

Thus the *general* action of the mont-Dore cure is clearly *antiarthritic*, since by stimulating and regulating the nutrition, increasing the activity of the organic oxydations, it effectually facilitates the uratic discharges and this to an extent apparent enough to attract the attention of the patients who call the second week of the cure, during which their urine shows the maximum of the exode of uratic principles, the « sand week ».

The *localised* action of the Mont-Dore cure is particularly *respiratory* antiarthritic, since it is the congestions, spasms, catarrhs and troubles of the respiratory organs from which the arthritic patients suffer, that are the most and best relieved.

The respiratory action, the functional therapeutic specialisation, is rendered as a *sedative* — less coughing, easier and less frequent expectoration, deeper respiration — and as a *decongestive;* sedation and decongestion are marked in the whole pulmonary apparatus, since organic and functional modifications can be appreciated from the nasal mucous membranes even to the pleural one.

If the interpretation of the effects obtained through the Mont-Dore drinking cure is difficult to give, their authentication is not so at all, for we no longer count the arthritic patients relieved, improved and cured at Mont-Dore.

The therapeutic results obtained by the Mont-Dore water, drunk, are very important; they give (considering the fact that the mineralisation is not very abundant) a new instance of the truth on which I insist so much, e. g. of how clinical results outweigh (in thermal medication matter) the chemical premises.

I could find here again, with what to justify certain velleities of *clinical* thermal classifications, that for the requirements of practice might appear preferable to the slight indications furnished generally by the composition of thermal waters.

It is possible that what experience teaches doctors to do *With* a mineral water should not matter to them more than its composition, which notwithstanding determines its classification ?

From a practical point of view of therapeutic indications, our art adapts itself more (excepting perhaps for strong alcaline waters, sulphurous waters, and those containing a large quantity of chloride of soda) to the results acquired in thermal polyclinics than to conjectures made from chemical analysis,

By what indication, for instance, can we augur (taking only into consideration the mineralisation of Mont-Dore), by what sign can we infer that the Mont-Dore treatment would perform wonders in curing respiratory troubles in arthritic patients? By what means can we tell that the action of the Mont-Dore water, which in virtue of its almost, specified affinities in the respiratory organs can determine in them, even when only taken by drinking, a slight substitutive anticatarrhal excitement, acting in its selective effects as a balsam drug ?

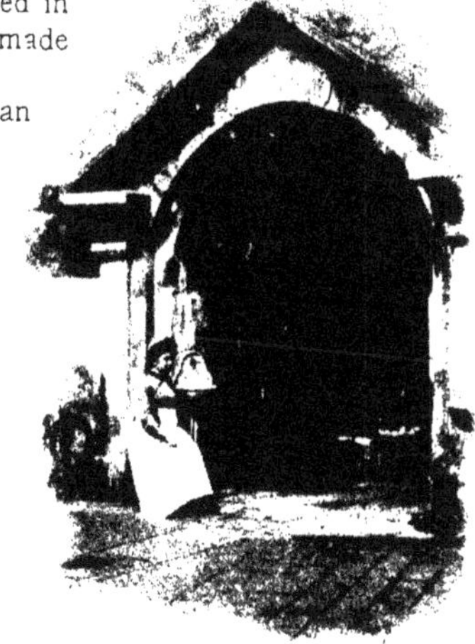

These special, not to say specific, results registered in the Mont-Dore polyclinic prove once more that it is the *reactive patient*, after all, who is the best to show the real value of the hydromineral specialisations.

*B.* — The **Hyperthermal baths**, which are one of the most curious and original processes of Mont-Dore, either general or partial — the former more employed than the latter — may be considered as one of the most important of the treatment.

But it is only one, you must remember, of the four essential processes of the cure followed by the many patients who visit the Establishment : I say four processes because to the drinking cure must be added the stimulation derived from the *Hyperthermal baths* (foot, hip, etc.) the *Inhalations* and the *High air cure*.

These hyperthermal hip-baths — in which one sits up to the waist during from 5 to 10 minutes at a temperature of 105 to 115 F., according to the abundance of water floving from the natural outlets at the bottom of each cabin, are *taken in running Water, spouting directly from the springs*, before the water loses any of its native properties (thermal, electric, chemical). They provoke on the patient at first, a slight vascular spasm, his pulse then becomes hard and frequent, then after the manner of artificial exanthema, an intense rubifaction appears over the whole of the parts emerged and immediately after, follows the perspiration of the upper part of the body.

Dressed again in his flannel costume the patient is taken back to his bed where he experiences a slight and not uncomfortable perspiration accompanied by a marked sensation of relief and then feels a manifestly increased freedom of breathing.

In cases of gout or rhumatism the repeated use of this powerful revulsive process might sometimes bring back, either immediately or later on, an arthritic or gouty flushing in the joints, or an exanthematic revival on the skin. In cardiopathic or nervous patients, this reaction might cause too much general excitement, which would not be exempt of danger.

The **Foot baths** taken also, at the spouts or in special tubs, as well as the **hand-baths** (prescribed when the former are counter indicated) form a revulsive process less intensive but more frequent and are made an almost general use of at Mont-Dore.

One can well understand how such stimulant and derivative processes, repeated daily, can both by nervous and vascular reactions, repercute from the periphery to the centre and from the centre to the periphery. One can understand how these processes must modify the nutritive and glandular activities as well as the functional of the respiratory apparatus whether it be the muccus membranes of the rhino-pharynx or of the bronchi, or the pulmonary circulation. One can understand how wonderful are their decongestive effects, proved every day by the results obtained during and after the cure, not only in the inflammation of the respiratory organs to which arthritic persons are so commonly exposed, but also in that of the air passages left after tuberculosis, measles, influenza, etc.

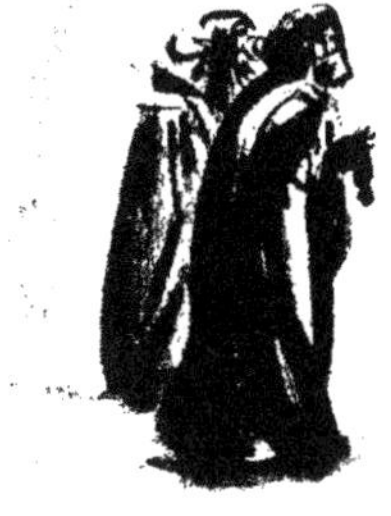

*C.* — The third process of the Mont-Dore medication is presented by **Inhalations**.

Thanks to the installation of the immense halls, heated at a temperature of 82, 86, 89° F., the process of inhalation is carried on in full ambulatory activity and not in the fixedness imposed upon in so many other Establishments, supplied only with inhalation cabins in which the small space only allows the patient room for sitting. During the twenty minutes, half hour, or hour that the patient remains in the inhalation rooms, he can sit, stand or walk about and talk, the inhalation being taken in the full operating of the organs, the patient experiencing, while he is walking or talking, quite a different mode of breathing to what he would where he to remain immovable before a vaporisator or sitting in a cabin too small for him to turn round in or move.

Contrary to theoretic previsions, the vapours caused by the boiling water contain in the inhalation rooms — besides a large proportion of $CO^2$, — clearly detectable and even dosable quantities of Si, Fe and As. This fact, which has been verified several times is due, according to the most plausible hyhothesis, to the sudden dislocation of the bi-carbonates in the boilers and to the mechanic carrying off of a few atoms of metals thus set free. It is very probable too that, from the effect of the reaction produced by these high temperatures, the Arsenic is spread in the medicinal fog partly at least in the form of volatile chloride; for the proportion of arsenic found in the vapours is relatively superior to the proportion of any one of the other mineral elements that have passed into the fog only by the mechanical carrying off.

The mineralisation of the medicamental fog is increased besides by the use of pulverisations effected on the progress of the vapour itself, which is thus loaded with metallic principles, in the same manner as the wind when it blows loaded with dampness.

Whatever the experiences and interpretations concerning the mineralisations of the atmosphere in the inhalation rooms may be, the luke warm fog inhaled in them is chemically medicinal and the clinical results, which are the principal object of our study, reveal in the most manifest manner its therapeutic effects.

At Mont-Dore, I was saying, the patients, while walking about in the large inhalation rooms breathe in the vapours that, descending to the very corners of the cells, fill up and impregnate every anfracture of the respiratory organs, from the meatus of the nasal cavities, from the sinus even, to the pulmonary infundibula. This damp, warm steam, loaded with mineral

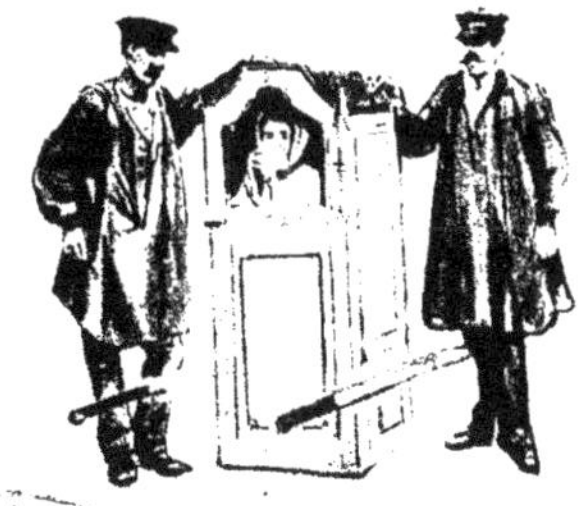



* *

elements, is spread throughout the aerial branches, imbibing, stimulating, and slowly flushing each part, increasing the activity o he bronchial secretions, provoking a kind of cleansing of the superficial endothelium and of the glandular epitheluims.

But the action of this steam on the respiratory mucous membranes does not appear to be simply *detergent*, manifesting itself by the fluidification of the secretions, by the expulsion of different catarrhal products or of fibrinous deposits and, amongst these, the saprophytic or pathogene flora, which lies on the surface of the crypts, pipes and alveoles. It is not only a similar action, from an antiseptic point of view, to that of any kind of purge destined to rid the cavity and walls of the digestive tubes mehanically of their anormal fermentations.

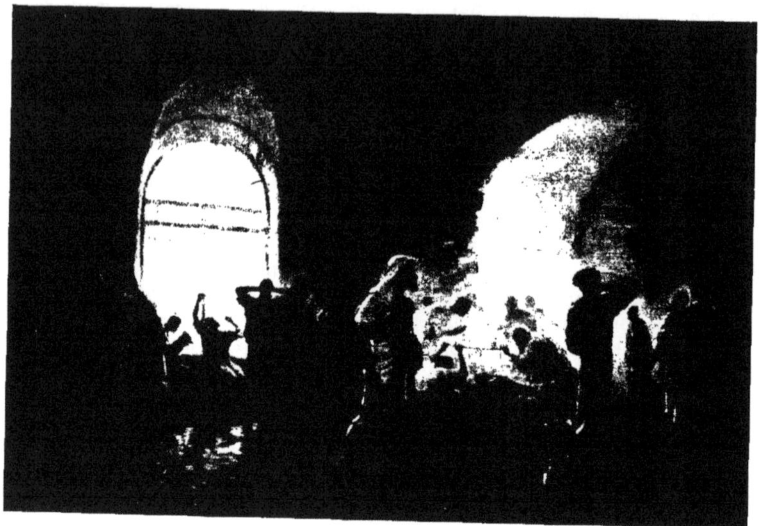

An inhalation room, from a painting by A. AUBLET. — " Cliché Braun, Clément et C^ie ".

It acts on the mucous respiratory membranes in a more lasting manner and, without attributing to it any *direct* bactericide effect (which however nothing appears to prove), we can compare the therapeutic action of the Mont-Dore water inhaled (like the action of the Mont-Dore water taken by drinking of which I spoke just now) and its stimulating action, *topically* fixed on the bronchial mucous membranes, to that which happens to the patients treated with balsam drugs and to the anti-catarrhal effects produced by these drugs through the respiratory mucous membranes.

The deep action that the Mont-Dore inhalations exercise on the pulmonary parenchyma, a decongestive and resolutive action that Clinics clearly show (as the action they exert on the diathesic ground) can be well understood, if one considers the important place the lymphatic tissues occupy in anatomy and in the physiology of the pleuro pulmonary branches as well as in the entire respiratory apparatus.

One conceives that the medicinal atmosphere on penetrating to the bottom of the glandular anfractuosities and of the alveoles, on renovating in each inspiration the deposit of metallic particles in the neighbourhood of the lymphatic lakes— that direct the cellular osmotic changes — modifies in them the molecular exchanges, urges on their elementary functions and stimulates their vitality.

If one takes into consideration (given the acuteness and intensity of absorption of the respiratory tubes) the length of time spent in the inhalation rooms on one side and the amplitude of the respiratory surface on the other, placed into contact with the vapours, we shall soon be convinced that in one hour's inhalation the absorption of the water through the pulmonary branches is equal to if not greater than the quantity taken each day by drinking.

The cure in the inhalation rooms has the great advantage of making the patients follow a kind of local treatment, acting like a topical medication as the vapours (endowed with organic affinities, if not with organic specification, lubrifying the mucous membranes topically urge these organs on to other nutritive activities, to other glandular secretions and functional activities, to other nervous reactions than those to which the rhinopathies, laryngopathies or bronchopathies, sequels to infectious diseases, such as measles, influenzan, tuberculosis etc. or manifestations of a constitutional state, had reduced.

If I insist on the inhalations as on one of the processes which each day occupy a more important place in the Mont-Dore medication, it is not only because many doctors attach great importance to them, through the sedation as well as the resolution of respiratory troubles, but also because most probably the process of inhalation acts partly in the same manner as the Mont-Dore water absorbed by drinking.

The immediate action of the inhalation, I have said, seems to be essentially *detersive* and *sedative*, calming like a topic and acting, by contact, on the nervous and spasmodic bronchial element.

To judge of the reality of the anti-spasmodic effect of the Mont-Dore vapours, it is sufficient to see an asthmatic patient taken into the inhalation room during his attack and to find him there again a few minutes afterwards expectorating easily and breathing freely. But do not mistake, this *immediate sedative effect* is not the only one; the *principal sedative effect* is that which is obtained after a certain length of time, sometimes after the second or third cure only, which consists in the definite suppression or at least in a persisting and very manifest diminishing of the frequency and intensity of the attacks.

To clearly perceive, at Mont-Dore, on the *decongestive* and *resolutive* action of the inhalations, we must follow from 5 to 10 days, a series of the really characteristic phenomenae on account of the order of their succession and of their paralellism. Let us take, for instance, a case of persisting tuberculosis with not actual pyretic reaction an old broncho-pneumonic focus, with a few cavernous lesions.

What the doctors at the Station observe, (and their experience on this point of view never varies), is firstly the modifying of the cough which becomes looser and less frequent, the expectoration previously painful, thick and of a yellowish green, becomes at the same time easier, paler, more abundant and aerated. In connexion with these modifications, the dull percussion noted over the congested part around the lesion becomes remarkably clearer, at the same time fine, dry rales are heard in the region where previously no sounds were audible, and these become progressively longer and moister; the patient from this moment, even before the expectoration has begun to dry up, observes the attenuation of panting in his walks and when ascending. So that this conjunction of changes, which are moreover accompanied by a marked improvement in strength, cannot leave any doubt as to the decongestive action of the vapours showing itself by the *fluidification of the secretions* and by the *return of the permeability* in the perilesional zone.

But neither is this all, for what you will often see for yourselves in your patients, at the end of the cure or from the first weeks following, it is that the expectoration diminishes and remains greatly lessened without ceasing to be whitish and discoloured, this is the recovering of the respiratory functions persisting in the perituberculous zones Often during the course of the year, you will remark in the entre of the softening part the indisputable signs of a fibrous or fibro-calcarous cicatrix, which is sometimes shown, independantly of a dry and permanent breath ng by an unexpected expectoration, in the full re-establishment of the general state, of one or two hemoptoic spittings surrounding a few pneumolithic fragments.

Moreover, whether it be a case of tuberculosis, less completely healed or a nevro-arthritic patient subject to bronchitis or to real relapses of congestion of the lungs, you will observe in either case that the habitual congestive fits will often be suppressed entirely or will at least become less frequent, less lasting, and certainly very much attenuated from the course of the first year.

It would be difficult to limit in this latter effect the part which belongs to the action of the inhalations and the part belonging to the water taken by drinking, but it will be sufficient to know that the effect is produced in certain patients who have not been submitted to the use of revulsive balneotherapy.

The action of these inhalations is therefore not only decongestive and sedative, acting as a poultice on the skin; but it seems also to have locally topically, a tonic, astringent, cicatrising ulterior effect, to judge from the benefit derived even by patients suffering from exulcerating affections of the respiratory organs, even in cases of open tuberculosis, provided that, on coming here, the patient, is not labouring under fever, provided that the specific affection is not, at this time, in a period of infectious activity.

III

You already know, gentlemen, the chief effects of the HIGH-AIR cure, which constitutes the fourth process of the Mont-Dore medication, so that I shall not remind you of them actually.

But we must not forget that — if the Mont-Dore water, when drunk, is anti-catarrhal and stimulating, if by the inhalations, combined with the muco-cutaneous revulsion, it is also sedative, decongestive, revulsive; all these results are obtained here, in a mountain resort and that in fact the Mont-Dore treatment is a **High-air, hydro-mineral, thermal cure.**

Here, this climatic element must not be considered only as a medicine for influencing on the general nutrition of the patient or for stimulating the appetite; here, the climatic element must be considered also as an element for influencing during the hydro-mineral treatment, the respiratory modalities (which are known to be different in mountain and plain). *To inhale and exhale the Mont-Dore vapours at a height of* 3500 *ft above the sea level*, forces on the patient a pulmonary excercise in no manner indifferent in the special purpose.

The respiratory movements increase in number only during the first days, they are then definitely enlarged; this accomodation of the pulmonary ventilation brings about a more complete expansion of the alveoli of all the pulmonary regions both of the upper as well as the inferior ones, causing a proper stirring up of the deeper regions and of the pleuro-pulmonary corticals in the medicinal atmosphere of the inhalation rooms; whence comes the treatment of the pulmonary and pleuretic consequences of various diseases, and as a definite benefit, at the end of the season, an increase of the pulmonary activity and a freer expansion of the lungs in the thoracic cage.

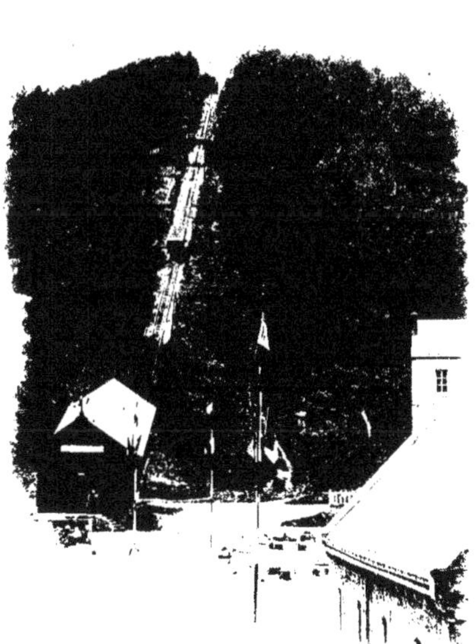

I very particularly insist on the very special association of therapeuties means, such as existing at Mont-Dore :

The broncho-pulmonary sedation and decongestion are not only caused by the derivation obtained from the hip and foot baths, the absorbing of the medical waters and vapours and the pulmonary massage (which is obtained through the breathing done in the inhalation rooms), but also by the mechanical, physiological, therapeutic properties in which the hydromineral medication is effected on the persons who breathe the air at a heighth of 3500 ft above the sea level.

Hence the reason why Mont-Dore, with her hygienic installation, her richness in hydro-mineral medicine and her complex accessories, including the funicular railway to the Capucin table-land, is the medication, if not specific, at least particulary special, marveilously adapted to persons affected in their *respiratory organs;* and this regards both : the patients who are only at their beginning of diathesic and professional irritations or congestions following infectious diseases (tuberculosis, influenza, measles, etc.). — just as well as those already victimed by localised inflammations.

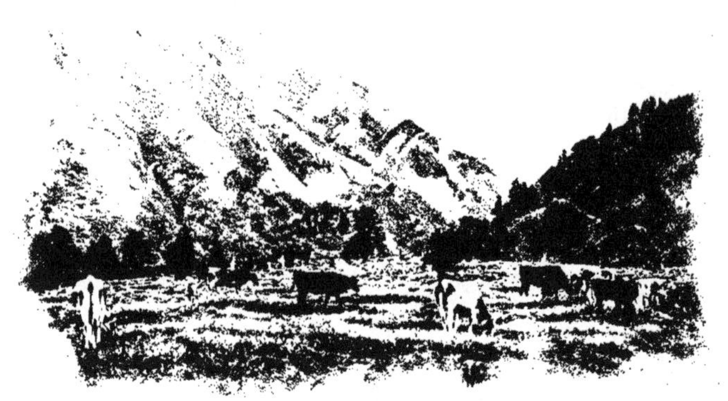

# Study of those Patients who have most benefitted by the Mont-Dore Cure

I

If we now attempt to determine which among our patients have given best proofs of the efficacity of the treatment at Mont-Dore, we must in the first place — in order to study the ORGANIC GROUND most adapted for benefitting by the effects produced upon the nutritive organs by the absorption of mineral water either as a beverage or by inhalation — remember what the clinical phisicians of the station have observed with regard to the initial uratic discharge during the « Sand Week »; and at the same time take into account what they teach us as to the therapeutic power of their treatment with regard to the functional respiratory disturbances presenting a *spasmodic or congestive character*. In this way we recognise, as do our colleagues, that the visitors to Mont-Dore must necessarily be recurited *above all* among patients showing **symptoms of the neuro-arthritic diathesis** either hereditary or acquired.

Further — on account of the sedative and resolutive effects of the Mont-Dore vapours on the tegument — we must mention here, amongst the forms of arthritis, its herpetic manifestations; without encroaching upon the domain of dermal diseases, we must mention among those who have cause to be grateful to Mont-Dore **certain sufferers** from **ezcema** in whom the cutaneous erruptions alternate or coincide with the congestions or spasms of the respiratory apparatus.

On the other hand — on account of the clearly anti-glucosuric effects of the mineral water absorbed — **certain diabetic** patients suffering from irritative affections of the respiratory organs, and threatened with or attacked by bacilli.

Finally — and I insist on this point, because, in the case of respiratory affections, if it is of importance to cure it quickly, it is of still more importance to prevent — we must note as having given proofs of the efficacity of the Mont-Dore treatment, **children** who, on account of **their personal** or **hereditary anticedents**, are subject to respiratory spasms, irritation or congestion, to which they are exposed by their arthritic diathesis, almost necessarily accidented by local infection from measles, grip, etc.

But it must understood that the Mont-Dore specialisation is two-fold : it is *diathetic*, and as such ANTI-ARTHRITIC ; and it is also *functional*, and as such efficacious in the treatment of RESPIRATORY affections.

As in the course of the cure the absorption of the Mont-Dore medicine reduces the quantity of azote in the waste, we recommend this station to patients suffering *at the same time* from **respiratory troubles** and **from insufficient assimilation of nitrogenous foods** — notably those which are *hypochlohydrous* — on account of the stimulating effect of the water absorbed upon the gastric secretion, an effect to which I called attention at the beginning of the lecture.

And it must be remembered that inhalation also, were it but by restoring the conditions of hematosis, contributes, with the other effects of the mineral water cure and of the High-air cure, to restore a considerable number of **patients** who are **"respiratorily invalids"** to a **general state of health in which the disturbances in the nutritive organs may be of an accidental order**, resulting from infection of whatever origin, or from various causes.

What was said just now with reference to the physiological action of the Mont-Dore treatment is a proof of its FUNCTIONAL SPECIALISATION, which attracts and with good reason, not only the diathetics, but **over-worked professionals**, and those suffering from troubles in the respiratory organs whether caused **by accident** or **by infection**.

It has been shown why and in what manner it is the treatment "par excellence" in so many cases of **respiratory catarrh**, especially of bronchial catarrh, It has been shown why the **irritations**, **congestions** and **spams**, (whether of nasal, pharyngitic, laryngitic or bronchial origin) from which so many persons suffer especially attacked with abarticular arthritis, are modified, diminish or even cease entirely under the influence of the treatment. It has been shown why public singers, orators, preachers, professors, lawyers, etc., etc., — in short all those whose *professional fatigue*, added in most cases to the effects of their arthritic diathesis, has produced catarrh of the first respiratory tubes — flock from day to day in greater numbers to Mont-Dore.

Patients whose table of respiratory symptoms is made up of nervous reactions, — a spasmodic cough, pulmonary attacks, or asthma (which was so justly described by our predecessors as an attack of the respiratory nerves) — should also go there to benefit by the anti-congestive, detersive dispersive and sedative effects of the cure.

*In reality* among the many persons suffering from fatigue of the vocal organs, among the few suffering from trauma of the lungs of the pleura, among those whose respiratory organs are weakened by intoxication, either exogenous (by ether, nitrous vapour, etc.) or endogenous (by fermentation of respiratory or digestive origin), among persons infected by grip, from rubeola or German measles, by tuberculosis or the mumps, there are many, certainly the great majority, who benefit by the treatment IN THE TWO-FOLD SENSE — FUNCTIONAL AND DIATHETIC.

As far as our *bacillary* patients are concerned, those among them who are born or who have become arthritic are most likely to benefit by the Mont-Dore treatment. This is not only because the peculiar mode of developement of their bacillosis is due to their arthritic temperament either hereditary or acquired, but also and especially because they react on the specific irritation (*trahit sua quemque voluptas*) according to their own erethic tendancies, by congestive or spasmodic excitement.

For these the Mont-Dore treatment, prescribed at the right time and repeated at intervals, is particularly efficacious, It reduces the number and intensity of the spasms and congestions, and helps the patient to calm and modify them; it limits the aeria of the groups of microbes so commonly associating in chronic diseases of the lungs; it helps to render permeable the pulmonary tissue, round about the injured part, and later on, to soften the scareous pleural adhesions.

THE AGE *even advanced* of our patients does not constitute a counter-indication — provided there is no pronounced angio-sclerosis — In persons over sixty who are subject to bronchitis, even those with a tendancy to a distension of the right side of the heart, the Mont-Dore treatment *followed prudently* and with daily supervision often obtain, together with a diminution or even the entire suppression of the attacks of bronchitis, the depletion of the right ventricle and the regularisation of the cardio-vascular functions, and the lasting disappearence of a malleolar oedema.

But it is not only in the case of adults that the Montdorian treatment may be applied to inflammatory, spasmodic and asthmatic affections of the respiratory organs.

**Children**, *young children even*, profit very much by the treatment which is applied to them here to get rid of the disorders left by certain forms of bronchio-pneumonia following upon grip, rubeola, or whooping cough; and it is the same thing in the case of the fits of asthma by which the descendants of arthritic people only too often betray, on approaching second chlidhood, the original taint. J. Simon used to send a great many of his little patients here and several of us, imitating his practice, find the Mont-Dore treatment very successful. In my opinion, it can never be applied too early to the children of neuro-arthritic persons, if it is desired to root out from the very beginning their functional respiratory troubles, and prevent them from developing into organic disease.

And I repeat here purposely, that whether it is a question of **children, of adolescents, of adults**, in whom organic or functional defects — primary recurrent or chronic, superficial or profound, simple or polymorphous — n the respiratory tubes testify to their diathetic condition, Mont-Dore should intervene *as a means of prevention* in order that the affection of the respiratory tubes may not pave the way for tuberculosis.

## II

This having been said, we can pass rapidly in review the LOCAL AFFECTIONS of the different organs of the respiratory system which benefit by the Mont-Dore treatment.

With regard to the **Rhinopharynx**, the Montdorian treatment is favourable to the *regression of the adenoid tissue* in children; in the case of soft and extended hypertrophy, in adults, it is only really efficacious after the surgical removal; and then it proves most beneficial in giving tone to the mucous membranes and preventing the too abundant increase of the glandular tissue. Among the neuro-arthritics, it is not those suffering from chronic not spasmodic hydrorrhoea, but those who are attacked with *congestive rhinopharyngitis*, with or without propagation towards the fallopian tubes, who have a chance of being cured at Mont-Dore. Those again who suffer from *hay-fever* or from *spasmodic rhino-bronchitis* are very often cured or sensibly improved, provided of course that the treatment is repeated for several years.

I will no more dwell on the benefits conferred at Mont-Dore by a tone-giving treatment on those suffering from *exhaustion of the* **Larynx** or by a sedative treatment on the neuro-arthritics suffering from *congestive attacks of the laryngo-tracheal tube*, from *nervous aphonia*, from *a spasmodic cough*, and, very often too, from *vertigo of laryngeal origin*. I will remind you that in patients suffering from *tuberculosis*, the larynx (were it simply on account of the diminution of the effects of this localised catarrh) also benefits by the Montdorian treatment, provided that the specific lesion of the organ is not yet profound, and provided that the infiltration is not of sufficient extent, to justify a fear of the possibility of an oedema in the glottis.

As regards the **intra thoracic** respiratory organs, the anti-congestive, sedative and revulsive treatment of Mont-Dore is absolutely made for all neuro-arthritics *subject to bronchitis*, whose conghing is dry, painful, coming by fits, irritating, whose expectoration is difficult, beady or viscous — for all rheumatic or gouty people, subject to *congestive tracheo-bronchitis*, dry *catarrh* of the bronchiae, or *congestion of the lungs, either erratic or recurrent.*

The treatment also suits all patients suffering from *bronchial catarrh* either *chronic or of frequent occurence*, and accompanied by *emphysema* — all those, young or old, whose pulmonary mucous membranes after being attacked by some infectious affection (influenza, pneumo-coccic diseases, whooping cough or rubeola) presents foci of *broncho pneumonia, permanent or recurrent, with or without symtoms of bronchial adenopathy* — all those who retain, near the top or near the bottom, remains of *pulmonary induration* all those again whose pleura has been affected and still presents symptoms of chronic inflammation, with or without lingering traces of effusion or of adhesion.

I said just that the Montdorian treatment is really beneficial with regard to **local respiratory tuberculosis**, when it is prescribed under favourable conditions.

One of these conditions has already been indicated by a single word in the letters of Sidoine Apollinaire on the waters of Mont-Dore, which he terms « aquae *phtisiscentibus* mirabiles ». Modern clinical physicians have succeded in defining its exact meaning without taking any thing from its comprehensive justice. It reminds us that the Mont-Dore treatment is directed not only against pre-tuberculosis or neo-tuberculosis hyperemia but also, in certain cases, against stages of pleuro-pulmonary bacillosis, which are anatomically and clinically more patient.

It is not because it is endowed with chemical properties actings pecifically or as antidotes, but because it is detersive, derivative, and anti-congestive, that the treatment creates circumstances less favourable to parasitic invasions; it is also because its topical action is scarring and at the same time has a power of resolvent, that it permits of regulating to some extent the procedure of curative sclerosis, and that it is the treatment for quite a variety of confirmed *sufferers from tuberculosis*, those even in whom the disease already begins to develope into phthisis.

An other condition of success is that the struggle against the disease must be undertaken *during an intermission of the specific pullulation and of the toxinic fever.*

When at the termination only of one of these agressive periods we confide certan of our tuberculous arthritic patients to our skilful colleagues at Mont-Dore that they may help them either to resolve the inflammation — post, peri, or para-tuberculous — or to soothe the parts round about the lesion, then the Mont-Dore treatment can produce startling results.

We have seen these cures, even in the case of certain of our patients suffering from phthisis and having been attacked in some degree by pulmonary consumption, provided that at Mont-Dore their doctor have tended them with a hand gloved in velvet, and provided of course that the organic ground put into contact with the Montdorian treatment was such as would permit of beneficial reaction, and of not offensive irritation.

With regard to this, it must be remembered that, by reason of its anti-congestive action, Mont-Dore — far from being dangerous in a case of *hemoptysis* (provided of course that there is no question of cavities with aneurismatic vessels or of neuropaths erethic to such a degree that the slightest physical or psychical stimulation brings on a hemorrhage) — generally succeeds in reducing the frequency and the intensity of the attacks of congestion.

Reserving for Eaux-Bonnes or for Allevard those suffering from a torpid form of tuberculosis, and for La Bourboule persons suffering from scrofular or from hereditary dystrophia; in whom the organic ground is highly susceptible to bacterial influence, and on the slightest provocation changes the fear into a reality, we must select those among the tuberculous patients who have an arthritic temperament and a congestive reaction, and send them here to Mont-Dore.

Basing my statements upon the results obtained under the same conditions carefully determined, I was able, at the Berlin Congress in May 1899, to oppose to the partisans of the uniform principle of treatment in a sanatorium for all forms of tuberculosis, the advantages of the application of the Brehmer principle in thermal and climatic stations, and, to extol with justice, among the most fortunate examples of these therapeutic associations, the ameliorations and cures effected at Mont-Dore upon certain tuberculous patients selected from among those suffering from congestive disorders and irritative lesions.

Of course — in view of these treatments by association, especially when prescribed for tuberculous patients – it is necessary to forewarn the patients against the prejudice that a regulation period of three weeks should be assigned to a thermal treatment; it is important to prepare for the possibility of prolonging the treatment according to circumstances and to intersperse the hydro-mineral treatment with periods of rest of more or less lentghy duration; rest and length of time being of the highest importance when treatments so active as those of MONT-DORE are in question.

It is also because of the happy results of the association of the mineral water treatment and of the altitude of Mont-Dore, that I have taught for so long, that I do not know a better or more desirable treatment for ASTHMATICS. That is provided that those called in nosography the true or essential asthmatics are not confused with the false asthmatics, really suffering from an attack of dyspnoea, induced by cardiopathy or nephropathy, which would be aggravated by a thermal treatment and by a great altitude. That is provided that there is really a question (as is generally the case) of larval bacilli, provided that the patient has symptoms showing that his asthma is due to spasmodic reaction brought on by a defective condition whether apparent or hidden, superficial or profound, of the respiratory organs.

It is in fact because of its sedative and dispersive inhalations and sometimes also because of its revulsive partial baths in conjunction with the climatic influence — that Mont-Dore merits its reputation of always being able to soothe and cure, at least temporarily, persons suffering from asthma; simply because true asthma, even when isolated, is generally a *function of bacillosis.*

I consider that the patient suffering from the asthma known as essential is subject to attacks of respiratory spasms, because he is affected by a *thoracic bacilleous thorn* which determines the localisation of the neurosis in the same way as does the nasal lesion so frequently incriminated.

As I speak of *larval forms*, it is not surprising that my opinion has been contested; but was not this opinion also contested formerly with regard to many other larval forms of tuberculosis, which are to-day clearly revealed in persons suffering from pleurisy, from athrepsia, from pseudo-typhoid, from sciatica, from spleno-pneumonia or from emphysema ?

The objection then should not be raised, that if such a veritable asthmatic subject after a career of repeated attacks of asthma, is formerly proved to be tuberculous, it is because the infection has seized upon him and rendered him tuberculous, although he is asthmatic ?

Since it has been necessary to admit as tuberculous, pathological conditions other than those wherein is manifested the nodule of Laennec, the larval forms of tuberculosis have taken their place in Phthisiology. The symptoms, however slight they may be, no longer permit the doctor to wait for the examination of the bacilliferous expectorations in order to classify from an etiological and therapeutic point of view, his divers patients whose purely clinical indications (together with family revelations) *savour* more or less of tuberculosis.

I am far, however, from under-rating the role which special or neuro-arthritic dyscrasia may play in the manifestation of pulmonary neurosis, when I teach that a tuberculosis spine, or a tuberculinous intoxication may exercise an important influence on it, were it merely as a determinative. If the tuberculosis does not manifest itself in the patients with the symptoms usual in the case of the classic embrys bacillosis, it is because the organic ground on which asthma generally manifests itself, partly explains the slow development of the tuberculosis. Matched in a neuro-arthritic temperament, the bacillosis attacks the convulsive dyspnoeic organs and for this reason certain neo-tuberculous arthritics are entered in the category of asthmatics.

Do we not know how many sclerogenous arthritics live as a rule in so called health with their tuberculous dependencies, wherever they may be situated ? Do we not the less gloomy prognostics to be formed in the case of all young women highly neuropathic or neurasthenic, in whom the tuberculosis, developing very, very slowly, tends rather to confine than to diffuse itself, exhausting them by the fits of coughing and of dyspnoea rather than by the fever, the bacilli proving in them infections in a remarkably slight degree ? Has not Pidoux already taught us to take into account the and specially slow peculiar progress of tuberculosis in a asthmatic subjects ?

Indeed the entire history of many asthmatics refutes the narrow conception formed by classic nosography of *true* asthma. I think that in this respect at any raten revision is necessary and that tuberculine (prudently employed as a probing injection) if used on a number of asthmatic patients might lead to many surprising revelations, in as much as the property of that form of tuberculosis, prevalent in neuro-arthritics, is to develope without fever and without expectoration, and therefore without affording an opportunity of having recourse to bacterioscopic examination.

It is the entire biography of many asthmatics, allowing at one stage or other of their existence the detection of their tuberculosis, that has led me to teach for so long that asthmatic persons ought to be regarded as tuberculous or, at all events, as suffering from a larval form of bacilleous localisation.

Without speaking here of other asthmatic subjects under my observation I state that, out of forty patients sent to Mont-Dore during this single season and personally known to me among my clientele or in my consultations, ten were asthmatic, some *apparently* tuberculous (I do not say phtisic after what I have just recalled to you as to the specific developement in these patients), the others *apparently* suffering from the action of bacilli. I say *apparently* because certain actual details of the symptomatology, together with the examination of their pathological history, permit me to affirm that in them, it is a question of larval bacilli.

The first thing found in them is the more or less complete list of the divers affections, the modality of evolution and grouping of which stamp them as neuro-arthritics. The second thing is the notation of infinitesimal shades in the palpation, the percussion and the auscultation of the thorax, shades which are all the more delicate in that they are generally masked by emphysema, especially at the periods nearly approached to the attacks. These shades in the tonality or elasticity to percussion, in the intensity of the vibrations, in the resonance of the voice and of the cough, in the fulness, the tone and the softness of the vesicular murmur, all these infinitesimal shades which are ascertained by a minute comparison of symmetrical zone are characterised by the *fixedness* of their seat. They are always found at the same points after congestive and spasmodic disturbances, just as they are found — with less difficulty generally in non-asthmatic neo-tuberculous subjects, after the artificial congestions provoked in the perilesionnal region by the use of iodures, which have been prescribed in my section for many years as a method for an early diagnosis of tuberculosis.

But if these stethoscopic indices necessitate minute and repeated investigations; if it is quite comprehensible that they may escape notice in an examination made during an actual attack or even during the period of acute emphysema which continues for a certain time after the attacks, even if it becomes impossible to seize upon them when permanent emphysema assumes a certain form or developement, — it is no less true that to one who studies the patient for a number of years, the suspicion is generally changed into a certainty by the occurence of some additional affection of a bacterial nature : in one case it may be the appearance of a sub-clavicular adenitis on the suscipious side or the revelation by the radioscope of a permanent opacity in the region of tracheo-bronchial ganglia; in another the coincodence of the beginning of the attacks with the bringing into activity of bacilli already noted or suspected which have been latent for several years; it is sometimes but more rarely the occurence of a baciliferous hemoptysis, occasioned by an accidental attack of congestion; but it is most often the slow yet progressive development of pleuro-pulmonary sclerogenous processus at the points primarily suspected of inceptive infiltration.

It is also — and that alas, frequently the manifestation of tuberculosis in direct filiation, for instance in persons living in close contact with asthmatic relatives, every where reputed to be in splendid health but for their asthma! In my lessons on larval tuberculosis I have often related heartrending stories on the subject. Such, among others, is that one of my sixty-year-old patients, who is now unmistakeably suffering from sclerous-tuberculosis in the upper part of the right lung, who has been charged from her youth with asthma, always reputed as *true*, and who, in what were apparently the most comfortable circumstances, contaminated three children and a maid who died of phthisis!

Finally the enquiry leads in some cases to the discovery of a specific contagion, clearly determined (on the occasion of a wound, for instance) and anterior to the beginning of the attack. This is why I insisted just now, on the necessity of inquiring *into* the entire patho'ogical antecedents of these patients, if one wishes to discover the very varied clinical circumstances which will completely explain the etiological diagnostic and to determine the real origin of the functional disturbances noted in asthmatic patients.

Concerning the false asthmatics, I should add that the medical men of this station are right in pointing out the persons in an advenced stage of Arterio-sclerosis who, notwithstanding all technical advice, present themselves at Mont-Dore as asthmatics and are astonished at their being ordered to leave the place, the more so that at the beginning of the cure they experience in the inhalation rooms, certain temporary improvement, because in the luke-warm atmosphere of the vapours their peripheric circulation becom for a time easier.

III

Although on reviewing the numerous kinds of illnesses in which the respiratory apparatus is called upon to benefit by the Mont-Dore cure, I have also many times pointed out those which could not profit by it, I think it would be useful to give you a few precise COUNTER INDICATIONS to the Mont-Dore cure.

It is important for a doctor, when he has a hydro-mineral station in view to which his patients may pay tribute, to have no less clearly before him the summary of the circumstances, strange or not, to the principal affections which render this choice inopportune.

He must not send to Mont-Dore either his *hepatopathic*, nor his *nephropathic patients*, for neither the treatment nor the climate would suit them, Neither must he send — excepting in cases of tracheo-bronchial adenopathy — any patient whose respiratory troubles might be imputable to a *tumour on the thoracic or cervical organs*, nor any one suffering from neoplasy, wherever it may be localised.

You will remember that a case of *pronounced angeio-sclerosis* would be badly placed here, if not on account of the thermal medication, at least on account of the altitude; and if in certain emphysematic bronchitic patients the Mont-Dore cure very efficaciously relieves the consecutive overworked state imposed on the right ventricule, it must not be forgotten that on the other hand neither the thermal treatment nor the High-air cure would be suitable to persons affected with *cardiopathy which was not entirely secondary or more especially one which might be insufficiently compensated*.

If in a general manner of speaking, it is among the neuro-arthritic patients affected with *functional or organic troubles of the respiratory organs*, that the clientele of Mont-Dore may be recruited, you will of course remember that not only the grave affections of the nervous system but also an *excessively exaggerated neurasthenic excitability* badly support the mountain climate.

As to pulmonary tuberculous patients, you will remember what I have said about the soil in which the grain germinates, and about the organic resistance and its fibro-congestive reactional modality.

# To sum up :

From what I have just exposed and the long developments attached to it, I wish you to retain the most important conclusions, concerning

1. Mont-Dore — one of the most *important hydro-mineral stations* in the department of Puy-de-Dôme, at over 3.400 ft above the sea-lavel — is rich in *hyperthermal, bi-carbonated, arsenical, silicious, ferruginious*, and *gaseous waters*.

2. The Montdorian treatment properly speaking (Drinking process, Hyperthermal cure consisting of baths in running water, Inhalation cure, intimately combined with the High-air cure) is a local and general medication, with *sedative, decongestive* and *reconstituent effects*

of which the DIATHETIC SPECIALISATION is ANTI-ARTHRITIC and of which the PRINCIPAL FUNCTIONAL SPECIALISATION is RESPIRATORY.

3. *To its primary or principal* FUNCTIONAL SPECIALISATION must be added a few secondary ones, regarding :

*a) Certain* **algic** patients — whose arthralgic, myalgic or neuralgic affections (notably the sciatic) occuring on the constitutional ground of arthritis, are relieved or healed by the decongestive and revulsive action of the hyperthermal hip-baths, just as well and sometimes better than by the effect of other divers cures of which the specialisation — such as at Néris, Bourbonne, Luchon, Bigorre, Aix-les-Thermes, Aix-les-Bains, for instance — seems to apply rather to the organic and functional disorders of the nervous system.

*b) Certain* stout and resisting **diabetic** patients, subject to congestive pharyngo-tracheal and broncho-pulmonary fits and in whom the Montdorian sedative and decongestive medication combats the respiratory affection and militates efficaciously against the invasion or the expansion of tuberculosis, lessening at the same time, in a very remarkable and persisting manner, the rate of glycosuria.

*c) Certain* **dermopathic** patients, whose vesicular arthritides alternate or coincide, especially in the form of eczematous slight and transient fits with congestive and spasmodic affections of the respiratory organs and of whom the Mont-Dore sedative and resolutive treatment can assure the recovery.

4. It is again on account of its FUNCTIONAL SPECIALISATION (and often even of its TWO-FOLD FUNCTIONAL AND DIATHETIC SPECIALISATION) that Mont-Dore claims very justly — among the pa-

tients affected with respiratory troubles either congestive or spasmodic — all those I have named as **respiratorily accidented persons** : the traumatised, intoxicated, infected, among whom I must reckon principally a whole category of persons subject to coughing, catarrhs, dyspneia, adenopathy, who for months have been suffering from the remains of whooping cough, rubeola, mumps, or grip, and in whom the resolutive decongestive and detersive medication soon heals their purely contingent respiratory infirmty.

It is often, too, due to its double specialisation, respiratory and antiarthritic, that Mont-Dore owes its just reputation of preserving certain patients predisposed to bacillose, of curing or greatly relieving *certain* **averated tuberculous persons** with congestive or spasmodic manifestations — so long as the stated counter-indications are severely born in mind in the very delicate selection of this kind of patients, to be sent here for this treatment.

Again it is, owing to its double specialisation diathetic and functional that this station succeeds so well with the **Asthmatic patients.**

5. Not only as a CURATIVE, because it stops the beginning evolution of their pharyngeal, laryngo-tracheal, bronchial and pleuro-pulmonary alterations but also as a PREVENTIVE, because it modifies, with their temperament, their aptitudes and their functional habits, and prevents their functional deviations from becoming organic — Mont-Dore is the station for **and children adolescents**; children who are so much exposed through neuro-arthritis, to congestive and spasmodic affections of the respiratory apparatus.

These thermal, *preventive, redemptive* cures, real instruments of puericulture necessary to avoid or correct opportunely, the defective functional creases that print themselves so easily and so deeply during the whole period of the growth of children, must be placed to the vangnard of therapeutic hygiene.

*
* *

*You will* remember, gentlemen, all the interest and extent of this therapeutic domain, so wonderfully perceieved by the gallo-roman empiricism, so justly maintained by the traditional medicine, so precisely confirme by the methodic observations of modern clinics; you will bear in min also the medical capacity of Mont-Dore, of which the functional specialisation includes, as a preventive no less than curative medicine, **every respiratory Arthritide.**

Without prejudice, without any exaggeration, nor false national self-pride, — you will retain that however resembling they may be in their mineral composition, however comparable they may be as a respiratory specialisation — no other waters in France or Abroad can be exactly substituted for these.

The Montdorian cure is unrivalled, because to the peculiar action of its organic hydro-mineral medicament — employed in all the living activity of its hyperthermal springs at the very outlets of the spouts themselves — it combines intimately the therapeutic effects with those of 3.446 ft of altitude. In this respect — excepting Wissembourg in Switzerland, of which the mineralisation, differs — neither Reichenhall in Baveria (1.542 ft) norinthe Taunus, Wiesbaden (382 ft), nor the Rhenish Prussian Kissingen (393 ft) nor Kreuznach (344 ft) nor in the dukedom of Nassau Ems (295 ft) can be compared to Mont-Dore.

All that I have said about its altitude and its hydro-mineral richness, all you have seen of its hygienic management and of its therapeutic installation, all you know of the progressive expansion of neuro-arthritis justifies the fame of Mont-Dore.

From this visit of the V. E. M. to the mineral waters of Auvergne, you will always remember that the station of Mont-Dore is not only one of the loveliest places in France, but that it is — on account of the importance of its diathetic and respiratory specialisation — one of the most powerful, and certainly one of the most compassionate (since it soothes, relieves and cures people suffering from respiratory troubles, who perhaps represent the greater part of the patients), stations in the world.

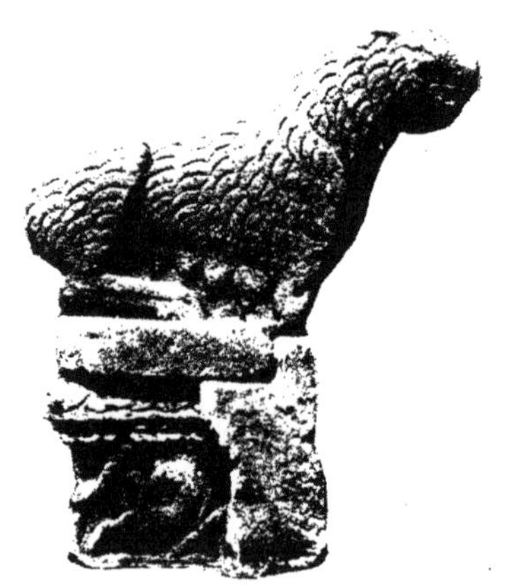

# INDEX



## THE MONT-DORE MEDICAMENT



## THE MONTDORIAN TREATMENT



## THOSE AMENIABLE TO THE MONT-DORE CURE

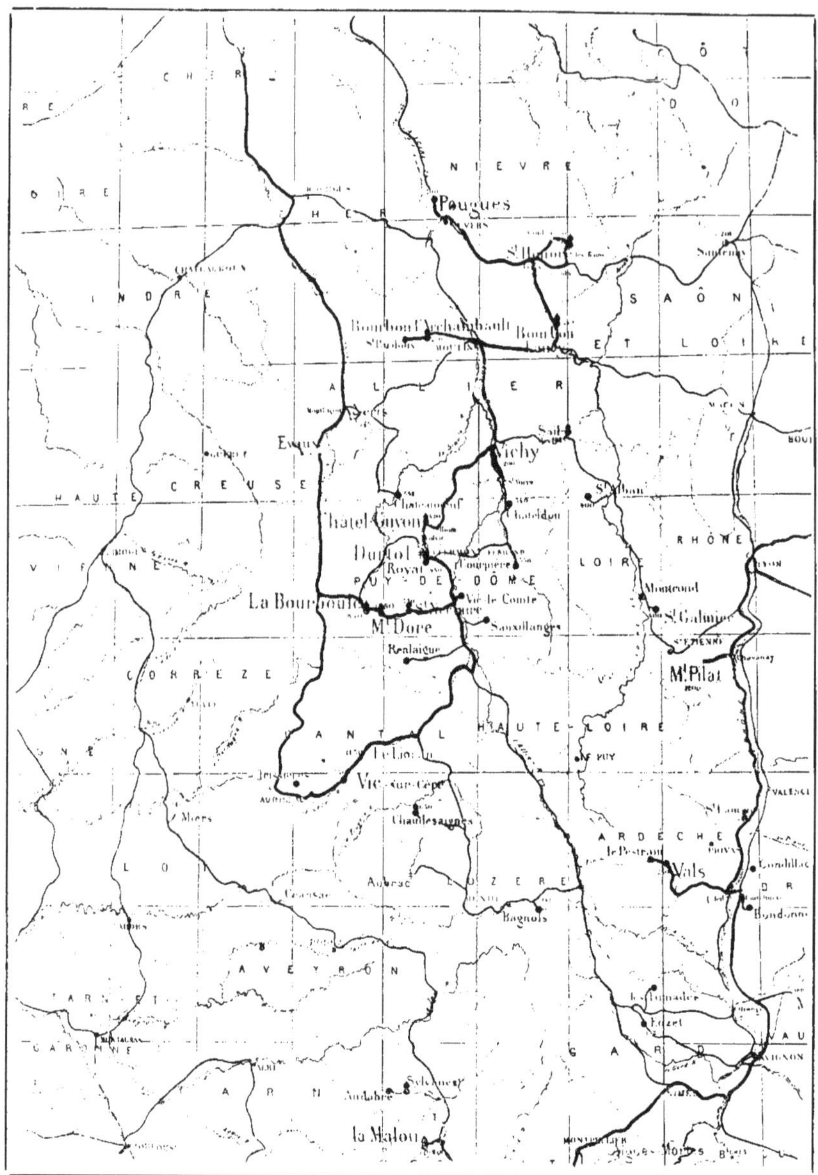


## ITINERARY OF THE V. E. M. IN 1904 TO THE STATIONS IN THE CENTRE OF FRANCE.

After the map of the Thermal, navy and climatic Stations of France, established by Professor Landouzy and Doctor Carron de la Carrière for the VOYAGES D'ETUDES MEDICALES.

PAPIER, GRAVURE, IMPRESSION
L. GEISLER, AUX CHATELLES,
PAR RAON-L'ETAPE (VOSGES).

www.ingramcontent.com/pod-product-compliance
Ingram Content Group UK Ltd.
Pitfield, Milton Keynes, MK11 3LW, UK
UKHW022003260726
13994UKWH00004B/1933

9 782329 378114